TREAT THE BLOODY PILES

Natural way to treat piles effectively

johny Einstein & Chatram Trivedi

Amazon kindle

Every one who shared their experience and methodology in this process of healing. You all are really great.

Take care of your food and it will take care of your body

JOHNY EINSTEIN

CONTENTS

FOREWORD

The book is detailed explanation about the discomfort which causes while passing the poop and long ignorant can create huge damage to the body. This book is an excellent expalnation and healing which some is facing for the longtime in his/her life.

INTRODUCTION

The journey of this book will take you to the concrete cause and its effective treatment of piles by following the daily regime and diet . which is as simple as drinking the water.

PREFACE

The aim of the book is to make every one strong enough to treat their disease naturally and effectively without any shyness as it prevails in every third person in the world.

PROLOGUE

This book required calm reading and thinking to understand the cause and in order to attain recovery .

TREAT THE BLOODY PILES

CHAPTER -1

Information about the piles

Piles, also known as hemorrhoids, are swollen veins in the lower rectum and anus. They can be internal, meaning they are inside the rectum, or external, meaning they are outside the anus. Piles can cause discomfort, pain, itching, and bleeding and can be caused by a variety of factors such as straining during bowel movements, constipation, pregnancy, and a low-fiber diet.

In severe cases, piles may require medical treatment, but in many cases, they can be managed through lifestyle changes, such as increasing fiber and water intake, reducing time spent sitting, and avoiding straining during bowel movements. Over-the-counter creams, ointments, and pads can also help relieve symptoms. If you think you may have piles, it's important to speak with a healthcare professional for a proper diagnosis and to discuss the best course of treatment for your individual case.

JOHNY EINSTEIN

CHAPTER - 2

One should not ignore piles

It is important not to ignore piles (hemorrhoids) because, although they are common and often not serious, they can cause a significant amount of discomfort and pain. If left untreated, piles can lead to more severe symptoms, such as bleeding, infection, or the formation of blood clots. In some cases, untreated piles can also lead to complications, such as anal fistulas (abnormal connections between the anus or rectum and the skin) or anal fissures (tears in the skin around the anus).

Ignoring piles can also lead to a delay in treatment, making it more difficult to manage the symptoms and achieve successful resolution of the condition. Additionally, ignoring piles may lead to the development of long-term complications, such as anal strictures (narrowing of the anus), which can impact bowel movements and overall quality of life.

For these reasons, it's important to seek medical attention if you are experiencing symptoms of piles, such as rectal bleeding, itching, pain, or swelling. A healthcare professional can diagnose the condition and recommend the best course of treatment for your individual case.

JOHNY EINSTEIN

CHAPTER - 3

Preliminary reasons of piles

There are several factors that can contribute to the development of piles (hemorrhoids): -

These are some of the most common factors that can contribute to the development of piles. However, it's important to keep in mind that not everyone who experiences these factors will develop piles, and that other underlying factors may also play a role. If you are experiencing symptoms of piles

CHAPATER - 4

Ayurveda in healing of piles

Ayurveda is a traditional system of medicine that originated in India more than 3,000 years ago. It is based on the concept that health and wellness depend on a delicate balance between the mind, body, and spirit. Ayurveda seeks to maintain this balance through a combination of personalized diet and lifestyle recommendations, herbal remedies, massage, and yoga.

Ayurveda recognizes three basic types of energies, called doshas, which are thought to govern the body and its functions: vata, pitta, and kapha. Each person is said to have a unique combination of these doshas, which determine his or her physical and mental characteristics and susceptibility to certain health conditions. The goal of Ayurveda is to identify the specific balance of doshas for each individual, and to use diet, lifestyle, and other interventions to maintain this balance and promote overall health and well-being.

Ayurveda is considered to be a holistic approach to health, and it views each person as a unique individual, rather than as a collection of symptoms or disease states. It emphasizes preventative measures and the use of natural remedies, and it seeks to address the root causes of disease, rather than simply treating symptoms.

While Ayurveda is widely used in India and other parts of the world, its use as a standalone form of medicine in the West is still considered to be complementary or alternative. It is important to consult with a qualified healthcare professional before using Ayurvedic remedies or making significant changes to your diet or lifestyle.

CHAPTER - 5

Importance of Ayurveda in treating piles

Ayurveda is an ancient Indian system of medicine that has been practiced for thousands of years and has a holistic approach to health and wellness. In Ayurveda, the focus is on maintaining balance and harmony in the body, mind, and spirit, which is believed to prevent disease and promote good health. Some of the key reasons why Ayurveda is important in treating various diseases, including piles, are:

CHAPTER - 6

Constipation creates the piles problems

C onstipation and piles are commonly related conditions, and one can often lead to the development of the other. In this context, let me explain how constipation creates the piles problem in detail.

Constipation is defined as having fewer than three bowel movements per week, and it can be caused by a variety of factors, including a low-fiber diet, lack of physical activity, and certain medications. When a person is constipated, they may strain during bowel movements, which can put extra pressure on the veins in the rectal area, leading to the development of piles.

Piles, also known as hemorrhoids, are swollen veins in the anus and rectum, and they can cause discomfort, pain, and bleeding. There are two types of piles: internal piles and external piles. Internal piles are located inside the rectum and are not visible, while external piles are located outside the rectum and are visible.

The straining that occurs during bowel movements due to constipation can cause the veins in the rectal area to become swollen and irritated, leading to the development of piles. Additionally, the increased pressure on the rectal veins can cause the veins to bulge out, leading to the formation of external piles.

Constipation can also make piles worse by causing the stools to become hard and difficult to pass. This can cause further irritation and swelling of the veins in the rectal area, leading to increased discomfort and pain.

Furthermore, a low-fiber diet, which is often associated with constipation, can also contribute to the development of piles. A diet that is low in fiber can cause the stools to become hard and difficult to pass, leading to straining during bowel movements and increasing the risk of developing piles.

In addition to the physical strain and increased pressure on the rectal veins, constipation can also lead to piles by causing emotional stress. People who suffer from chronic constipation may become frustrated and stressed, which can increase their risk of developing piles. This is because stress and anxiety can cause the body to produce hormones that increase pressure in the rectal veins, leading to the development of piles.

CHAPTER - 7

Emotional stress creates piles problem

Emotional stress and piles are commonly related conditions, and one can often lead to the development of the other. In this context, let me explain how emotional stress creates the piles problem in detail.

Emotional stress refers to feelings of tension, anxiety, and pressure that can be caused by a variety of events or circumstances, such as work, relationships, or financial problems. When a person experiences emotional stress, their body reacts in a number of ways that can increase their risk of developing piles.

One of the ways that emotional stress can contribute to the development of piles is by causing the body to produce hormones such as cortisol and adrenaline. These hormones increase the pressure in the veins in the rectal area, leading to the development of piles. Additionally, emotional stress can cause the muscles in the rectal area to tense up, further increasing the pressure on the veins and increasing the risk of developing piles.

Emotional stress can also contribute to the development of piles by causing changes in bowel movements. People who are under stress often experience changes in their digestive system, including constipation, diarrhea, or alternating between the two. Constipation, in particular, can increase the risk of developing piles because it can cause the stools to become hard and difficult to pass, leading to straining during bowel movements.

Furthermore, emotional stress can cause changes in eating habits, which can also increase the risk of developing piles. People who are under stress may overeat, undereat, or eat unhealthy foods, which can contribute to constipation and increase the risk of developing piles.

In addition to the physical effects, emotional stress can also contribute to the development of piles by causing psychological stress and anxiety. People who are under stress may become frustrated, anxious, and depressed, which can increase their risk of developing piles. This is because psychological stress can cause the muscles in the rectal area to tense up, further increasing the pressure on the veins and increasing the risk of developing piles.

Emotional stress and piles are closely related conditions, and one can often lead to the development of the other. Emotional stress can contribute to the development of piles by increasing the pressure in the veins in the rectal area, causing changes in bowel movements, and leading to changes in eating habits. Additionally, emotional stress can cause psychological stress and anxiety, which can also increase the risk of developing piles.

Therefore, it is important to manage emotional stress to help prevent the development of piles. This can be done by practicing stress management techniques, such as deep breathing, meditation, and exercise, and by eating a healthy and balanced diet. If you are already suffering from piles, managing emotional stress can help reduce your symptoms and improve your overall quality of life.

CHAPTER - 8

Fibrous diet in treating piles

A high-fiber diet is an essential component in the treatment of piles, also known as hemorrhoids. Hemorrhoids are swollen veins in the rectal area that can cause discomfort, pain, and itching. The importance of a fibrous diet in treating piles lies in its ability to regulate bowel movements and prevent constipation, which is one of the main causes of piles.

Fiber is the indigestible part of plant-based foods, such as fruits, vegetables, whole grains, and legumes, that helps regulate bowel movements. It helps to soften stools, making them easier to pass, and reduces the risk of constipation. When stools are soft, they are less likely to cause straining during bowel movements, which can put pressure on the veins in the rectal area and lead to the development of piles.

In addition to preventing constipation, a high-fiber diet can also help to reduce the symptoms of existing piles. Fiber helps to absorb water and add bulk to the stools, making them easier to pass and reducing the risk of further irritation to the rectal area. This, in turn, can help to reduce symptoms such as pain, itching, and bleeding.

Fiber also has a number of other health benefits, including reducing the risk of heart disease, stroke, and some types of cancer. It can also help to regulate blood sugar levels and lower cholesterol levels. In addition, fiber-rich foods tend to be low in calories and high in nutrients, making them a healthy addition to any diet.

When it comes to incorporating fiber into your diet, it is important to do so gradually to avoid digestive discomfort, such as bloating and gas. Start by incorporating small amounts of high-fiber foods into your diet and gradually increasing your intake as your body adjusts. Some good sources of fiber include fruits, such as berries, apples, and pears, vegetables, such as spinach, carrots, and peas, whole grains, such as brown rice, whole wheat bread, and oatmeal, and legumes, such as lentils, chickpeas, and black beans.

It is also important to drink plenty of water when incorporating a high-fiber diet into your diet. Fiber needs water to work effectively, and if you do not drink enough water, the fiber can actually make constipation worse. Aim to drink at least 8 glasses of water a day to help keep your stools soft and regulate your bowel movements.

A high-fiber diet is an essential component in the treatment of piles. Fiber helps to regulate bowel movements, prevent constipation, and reduce the symptoms of existing piles. By incorporating fiber-rich foods into your diet and drinking plenty of water, you can help to improve your overall health and reduce your risk of developing piles. If you are already suffering from piles, incorporating a high-fiber diet into your daily routine can help to reduce your symptoms and improve your quality of life.

CHAPTER - 9

Diet chart for Piles

Diet chart for high fibrous food for breakfast, lunch and dinner

a sample diet chart for a high-fiber diet, including breakfast, lunch, and dinner:

Breakfast:

Lunch:

Dinner:

Snacks:

vegetarian Diet chart for high fibrous food for breakfast, lunch and dinner

Breakfast:

Lunch:

Dinner:

Snacks:

Remember, it is important to drink plenty of water when incorporating a high-fiber diet into your diet. Aim to drink at least 8 glasses of water a day to help keep your stools soft and regulate your bowel movements.

It is also important to note that everyone's needs are different and you may need to adjust the amounts and types of fiber-rich foods to suit your individual needs. If you experience digestive discomfort, such as bloating or gas, you may need to reduce your fiber intake and increase your water consumption. Additionally, if you have any existing health conditions, you should consult with your doctor or a registered dietitian before making any major changes to your diet.

CHAPTER - 10

Avoiding of spicy and fatty
food in treating piles

Spicy and fatty foods can have a significant impact on the health of the digestive system and are often discouraged for people suffering from hemorrhoids or piles. These foods can contribute to the development of piles and make existing piles symptoms worse. In this article, we will discuss the reasons why spicy and fatty foods should be avoided in treating piles, and provide some tips on how to maintain a healthy diet to manage this condition.

Why Should Spicy and Fatty Foods be Avoided in Treating Piles?

Avoiding spicy and fatty foods is an important aspect of treating piles. These foods can be irritating to the digestive system and make existing piles symptoms worse. To manage piles symptoms, it is important to maintain a healthy diet.

JOHNY EINSTEIN

CHAPTER - 11

Importance of sitz bath in treating piles

Sitz baths are a type of warm-water bath that are commonly recommended for the treatment of hemorrhoids (also known as piles). A sitz bath can provide relief from the discomfort and pain associated with hemorrhoids, and can also help to promote healing. In this article, we will discuss the importance of sitz baths in treating piles.

What are Hemorrhoids? Hemorrhoids are swollen veins in the anus and rectum that can cause discomfort and pain. There are two types of hemorrhoids: internal and external. Internal hemorrhoids are located inside the rectum, while external hemorrhoids are found outside the anus. Hemorrhoids are often caused by increased pressure in the veins in the rectal area, which can be due to factors such as constipation, straining during bowel movements, pregnancy, obesity, and prolonged sitting.

What is a Sitz Bath? A sitz bath is a shallow bath that is specifically designed to soothe and clean the rectal and genital areas. The term "sitz" comes from the German word "sitzen," which means "to sit." The bath is taken while sitting in a tub that is specifically designed for the purpose, or in a regular bathtub with the bottom part filled with warm water.

Benefits Of Sitz Baths For Hemorrhoids:

How To Take A Sitz Bath:

It is important to note that sitz baths should not be taken as a replacement for other treatments for hemorrhoids, such as fiber-rich foods, increased water consumption, and over-the-counter creams and ointments. Sitz baths should be used in conjunction with other treatments,

Sitz baths are an effective and non-invasive treatment option for hemorrhoids. The warm water can provide relief from pain and discomfort, promote healing, cleanse the rectal area, increase circulation, and relieve itching and irritation. If you are suffering from hemorrhoids, incorporating sitz baths into your treatment plan can be a valuable part of it.

Recommendation :- Every time you go to bathroom to pass the stool , take the warm water sitz for at least 10 minutes to get maximum results effectively.

CHAPTER - 12

Aloe Vera use in piles treatment

Aloe Vera is a natural plant with a long history of use in traditional medicine. It has a wide range of health benefits, including its ability to treat hemorrhoids or piles. In this article, we will discuss the benefits of using Aloe Vera for the treatment of piles and how it can be used for permanent relief.

How Does Aloe Vera Help in Treating Piles?

How To Use Aloe Vera For Treating Piles:

Aloe Vera is a natural plant with a wide range of health benefits, including its ability to treat hemorrhoids or piles. Its anti-inflammatory, moisturizing, and healing properties can help to relieve discomfort and promote healing in the rectal area. To get the best results, it is important to use pure, organic Aloe Vera products and speak with a healthcare professional before starting any new treatment regimen. While Aloe Vera can help to manage symptoms of piles, it is not a permanent cure. To achieve permanent relief, it is important to address the underlying causes of hemorrhoids, such as constipation and increased pressure in the veins in the rectal area.

JOHNY EINSTEIN

CHAPTER - 13

*Triphla Churna ayurvedic medicine
in piles treatment*

Triphala is a popular ayurvedic medicine that has been used for centuries in the treatment of a variety of health conditions, including piles or hemorrhoids. Triphala is a combination of three fruits - amla, haritaki, and bibhitaki - that are rich in antioxidants and other beneficial compounds.

How Does Triphala Help in Treating Piles?

How to Use Triphala for Treating Piles:

Oral Supplement: Triphala can be taken orally in the form of a supplement or powder. The best way to take is one full spoon with warm water after dinner before sleep. Also It is important to speak with a healthcare professional before starting any new supplement regimen if you are taking any other specific medicine although ayurvedic medicines or churna (Powder) have no side effect.

CHAPTER - 14

Psyllium husk in treating of piles

Psyllium husk is a type of soluble fiber that is commonly used in the treatment of various digestive conditions, including hemorrhoids or piles. This versatile fiber is derived from the seeds of the Plantago ovata plant and has been used for centuries in traditional medicine to promote digestive health.

How Does Psyllium Husk Help in Treating Piles?

psyllium husk is a versatile and effective fiber that can be used in the treatment of hemorrhoids or piles. Its laxative, anti-inflammatory, and digestive health properties can help to relieve discomfort and promote healing in the rectal area. To get the best results, it is important to use high-quality psyllium husk products and speak with a healthcare professional before starting any new treatment regimen. While psyllium husk can help to manage symptoms of piles, it is not a permanent cure. To achieve permanent relief, it is important to address the underlying causes of hemorrhoids, such as constipation and increased pressure in the veins in the rectal area. In addition to psyllium husk, a healthy diet that is rich

Key rule for in healing of piles is never put the pressure while passing on the stools (Poop) in the toilet

www.ingramcontent.com/pod-product-compliance
Lightning Source LLC
Chambersburg PA
CBHW080913220526
45467CB00021BA/3394